CARNIVORE DIET COOKBOOK FOR WOMEN OVER 60

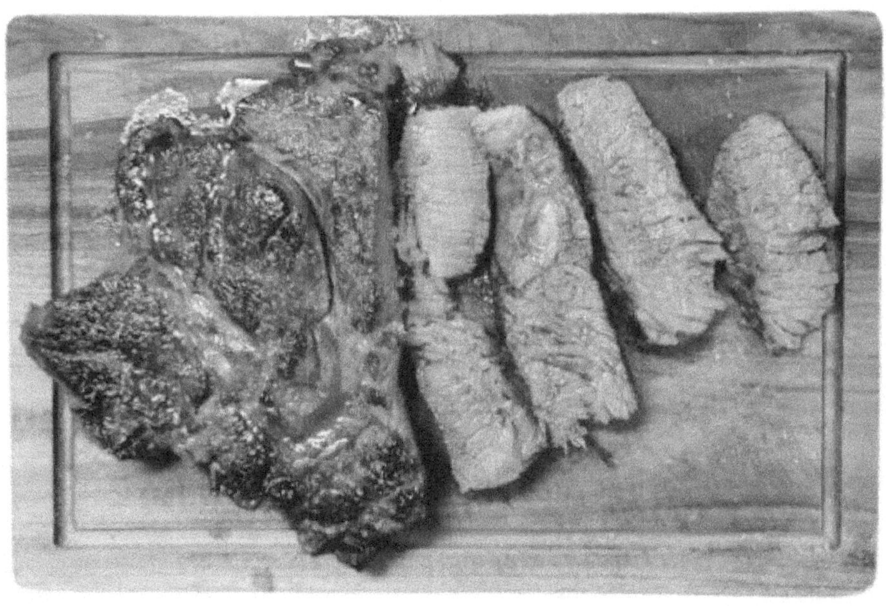

ALEX PEACHEY

DISCLAIMER

The content within this book reflects my thoughts, experiences, and beliefs. It is meant for informational and entertainment purposes. While I have taken great care to provide accurate information, I cannot guarantee the absolute correctness or applicability of the content to every individual or situation. Please consult with relevant professionals for advice specific to your needs.

TABLE OF CONTENTS

INTRODUCTION

Hello there, fellow culinary explorers! I'm Chef Alex Peachey, and I'm beyond excited to take you on a gastronomic journey that has not only transformed my life but promises to transform yours too. Buckle up as I share my personal odyssey from a childhood of diverse eating habits to becoming a fervent advocate of the carnivore lifestyle.

Growing up, I wasn't the quintessential carnivore. In fact, vegetables and fruits were the superheroes on my plate, and meat was often relegated to the sidekick role. My taste buds danced with the vibrant flavors of an array of foods, and the concept of a carnivore diet was as foreign to me as intergalactic travel.

Fast forward a few decades, and life had taken its toll. The scale groaned under the weight of my unhealthy eating habits, and the mirror echoed my struggles. The once vibrant and energetic me was now bogged down by excess weight, sluggishness, and a feeling of discontent. It was at this juncture that the carnivore diet entered my life like a culinary superhero, ready to rescue me from the clutches of unhealthy living.

The transition wasn't an overnight affair. I was a chef with a penchant for experimenting in the kitchen, and my culinary curiosity led me to explore the carnivore lifestyle. Skepticism mingled with excitement as I embarked on this uncharted culinary adventure. Questions danced in my mind: Could this diet really be the key to shedding unwanted pounds? What about the vitamins and nutrients I'd be missing from fruits and vegetables? Would I feel satisfied and energetic, or would I be left craving the colorful plates of my past?

The answers revealed themselves gradually but convincingly. As I embraced the carnivore diet, the excess weight melted away like snow under the warm sun. It wasn't just a physical transformation; my energy levels soared, and a renewed sense of vitality swept through me. The carnivore lifestyle became a revelation, a secret ingredient that had been missing from my culinary repertoire all along.

Why did the carnivore diet work so effectively? It's a question I asked myself as I delved into the science behind this dietary approach. The benefits unfolded like a well-crafted recipe. This diet, rich in high-quality meat and animal-based products, provides essential nutrients in their most bioavailable form. The simplicity of consuming nutrient-dense foods directly from the animal kingdom eliminates the guesswork often associated with complex dietary plans.

Allow me to pose a question to you, dear reader: How many diets promise you weight loss without counting calories or measuring portions? The carnivore diet, a beacon of simplicity in a world drowning in dietary advice, allows you to eat until satisfied. It's a liberating feeling, breaking free from the shackles of restrictive diets and embracing a lifestyle that nourishes both body and soul.

Now, let's talk about the dangers lurking in our modern eating habits. The shelves of grocery stores are laden with processed, sugar-laden concoctions masquerading as food. We're bombarded with choices that lead us down a path of inflammation, weight gain, and myriad health issues. The carnivore diet, in contrast, is a return to the basics. It's a recalibration, a way to reset your body and mind.

As a seasoned chef with over 25 years of experience, I've witnessed the transformative power of culinary choices. The recipes within this cookbook aren't just a collection of dishes; they're a celebration of health, vitality, and the joy of savoring every bite. Each recipe is a brushstroke on the canvas of your well-being, carefully crafted to bring you the benefits of the carnivore lifestyle without compromising on flavor.

But why should you choose this cookbook? Allow me to share my perspective. This isn't just a collection of recipes; it's a guide to a healthier, happier you. Whether you're a seasoned carnivore or a curious beginner, these recipes are designed to tantalize your taste buds and nurture your body. The advantage lies in the simplicity of carnivore cooking – fewer ingredients, less fuss, and more time for the things that truly matter.

In this cookbook, I've poured my heart and soul into each recipe, drawing on years of research, experimentation, and a love for the culinary arts. From succulent meat skewers to savory organ meat creations, these recipes offer a diverse and delicious array of options. It's not just a cookbook; it's a roadmap to a new chapter in your culinary journey.

As you embark on this carnivore culinary adventure, ask yourself: What if the key to a healthier, more vibrant you is right here, within the pages of this cookbook? What if the simplicity of a carnivore lifestyle could be the secret ingredient missing from your life?

Let's turn the page together and savor the flavors of a new beginning. Welcome to a world where taste meets transformation, and every bite is a step toward a healthier, more fulfilling life. Cheers to the journey ahead – may it be as delectable as the dishes you're about to discover!

Contact the Author

Thank you for reading my book! I would love to hear from you, whether you have feedback, questions, or just want to share your thoughts. Your feedback means a lot to me and helps me improve as a writer.

Please don't hesitate to reach out to me through

contactalexpeachey@gmail.com

I look forward to connecting with my readers and appreciate your support in this literary journey. Your thoughts and comments are valuable to me.

CARNIVORE DIET COOKBOOK FOR BEGINNERS

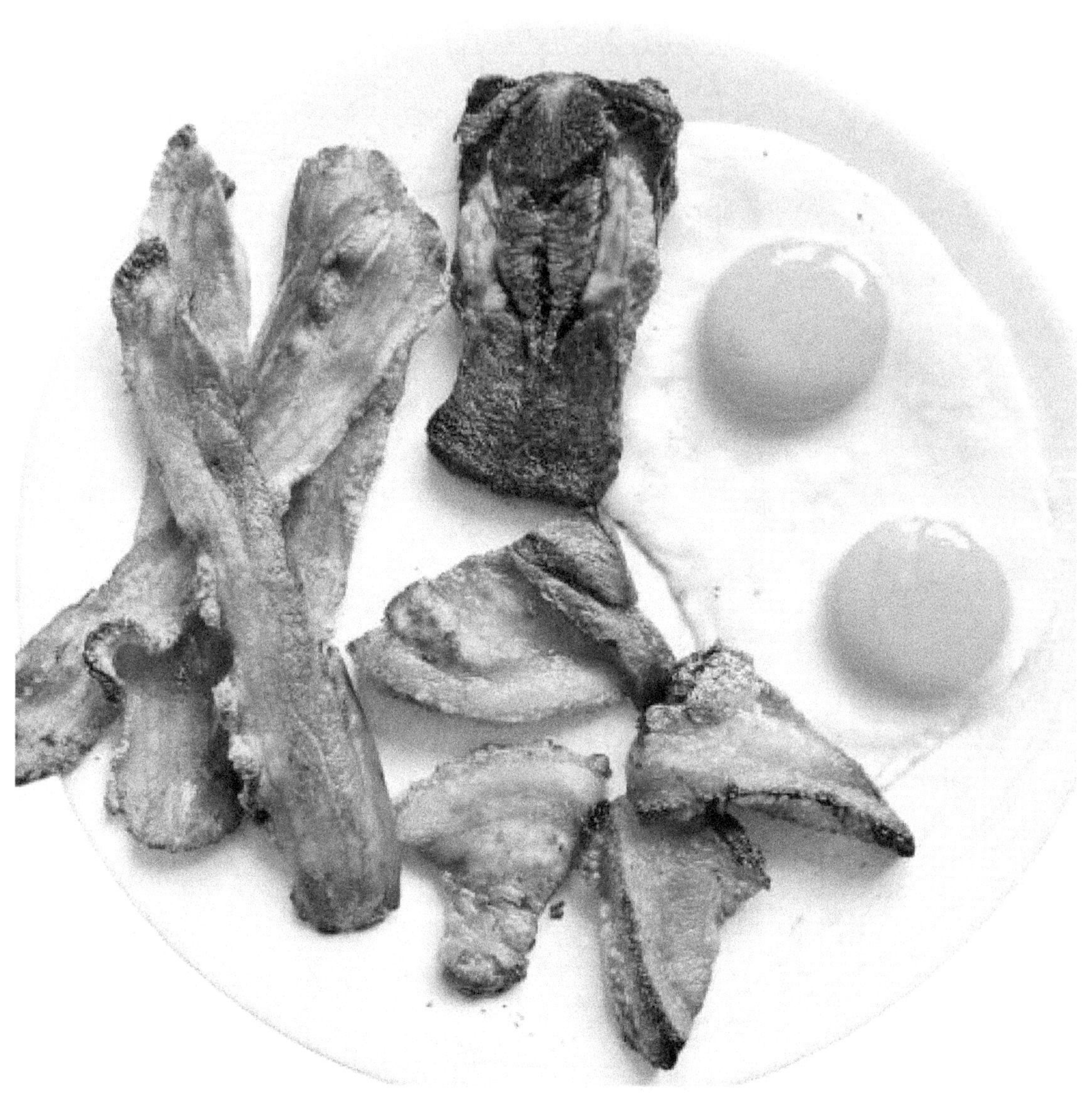

CHAPTER 1

UNDERSTANDING THE CARNIVORE DIET

The Carnivore Diet, characterized by its exclusive reliance on animal products, has generated considerable interest, prompting a closer examination of its scientific foundations. In this comprehensive exploration, we delve into the intricacies of the Carnivore Diet's science, its potential advantages for women over 60, and a nuanced exploration of common concerns associated with this distinctive dietary approach.

The Science Behind the Carnivore Diet:

1. **Nutrient Density and Bioavailability:**

   - Animal products, such as meat, organ meats, and eggs, are renowned for their superior nutrient density and bioavailability. The Carnivore Diet capitalizes on these characteristics, providing easily absorbable forms of essential nutrients like iron, zinc, and B vitamins, which are crucial for maintaining optimal health, particularly in aging individuals.

2. **Ketosis and Metabolic Flexibility:**

   - The low-carbohydrate nature of the Carnivore Diet induces ketosis, a metabolic state where the body utilizes ketones derived from fats for energy. This shift in metabolic flexibility may not only aid in weight management but also hold potential benefits for cognitive function and energy stability, particularly in the context of age-related metabolic changes.

3. **Inflammation Reduction and Autoimmune Implications:**

- Emerging research suggests that the exclusion of certain plant-based compounds in the Carnivore Diet may contribute to reduced inflammation. For women over 60, this anti-inflammatory potential holds promise in addressing age-related inflammatory conditions and potentially mitigating autoimmune responses.

Benefits for Women Over 60:

1. **Enhanced Nutrient Absorption:**

   - The Carnivore Diet's emphasis on animal-based foods, known for their digestibility, can be especially advantageous for women over 60 who may face challenges in nutrient absorption. The absence of anti-nutrients commonly found in plants may further optimize the absorption of essential nutrients critical for overall health.

2. **Preservation of Lean Muscle Mass:**

   - Protein, a cornerstone of the Carnivore Diet, plays a pivotal role in preserving lean muscle mass. As women age, maintaining muscle becomes increasingly vital for functional independence. The high-quality protein from animal sources aids in preserving muscle integrity, contributing to overall physical well-being.

3. **Hormonal Balance and Menopausal Support:**

   - The diet's impact on hormonal balance, particularly through increased fat intake, has implications for women navigating menopause. Proponents suggest that the Carnivore Diet may alleviate symptoms such as mood swings and hot flashes, potentially providing a natural approach to hormonal management during this life stage.

Addressing Common Concerns:

1. **Comprehensive Nutrient Intake:**

    - Critics often raise concerns about potential nutrient deficiencies on the Carnivore Diet. However, advocates emphasize the importance of variety within the animal kingdom, encouraging the consumption of different cuts of meat, organ meats, and incorporating fish to ensure a comprehensive nutrient profile.

2. **Adaptation of the Digestive System:**

    - The absence of dietary fiber from plant sources raises questions about its impact on digestive health. Proponents argue that the human digestive system is adaptable and can thrive on a lower-fiber diet. Furthermore, the inclusion of organ meats, which provide essential nutrients and support gut health, contributes to a holistic approach.

3. **Sustainable Sourcing Practices:**

    - Environmental sustainability concerns associated with meat production are acknowledged. To address this, proponents of the Carnivore Diet advocate for responsible sourcing, emphasizing the importance of choosing ethically raised and sustainably produced meats to minimize the environmental impact.

4. **Long-Term Considerations and Individualized Approaches:**

- While ongoing research explores the long-term effects of the Carnivore Diet, it is essential for individuals, especially women over 60, to approach this dietary choice with caution. Consulting healthcare professionals can provide personalized guidance, considering individual health conditions, and ensuring the diet aligns with specific needs and goals.

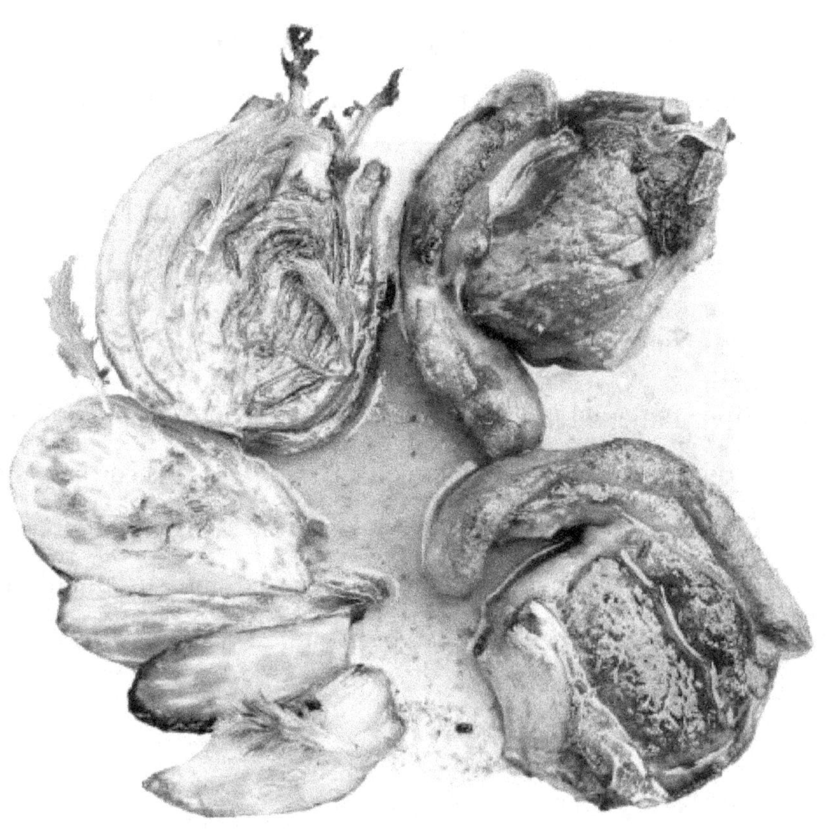

CHAPTER 2

GETTING STARTED

Embarking on the Carnivore Diet requires thoughtful planning and preparation, especially for women over 60 seeking to optimize their health. This cookbook will help you get started by assessing your health goals, highlighting essential items for your carnivore kitchen, and providing a comprehensive grocery shopping guide tailored to the unique needs of women in this demographic.

1. **Assessing Your Health Goals:**

   - Before diving into the Carnivore Diet, take the time to assess your health goals. Whether you're aiming for weight management, improved energy levels, or specific health outcomes, having a clear understanding of your objectives will help tailor your approach and track progress effectively.

2. **Consulting Healthcare Professionals:**

   - Given the unique nutritional needs of women over 60, it's crucial to consult with healthcare professionals before starting any new diet. They can provide personalized advice, considering factors such as existing health conditions, nutrient requirements, and potential challenges associated with the Carnivore Diet.

Kitchen Essentials for Carnivore Cooking:

1. **Quality Meat Sources:**

   - Invest in high-quality meat sources, including grass-fed beef, pasture-raised poultry, lamb, and wild-caught fish. These form the foundation of the Carnivore Diet, providing essential nutrients in their most bioavailable forms.

2. **Organ Meats:**

   - Incorporate organ meats like liver, heart, and kidney into your diet. These nutrient-dense organs offer a wide range of vitamins and minerals, contributing to a well-rounded nutritional profile.

3. **Saturated Fats:**

   - Include sources of healthy saturated fats, such as butter, ghee, and tallow, to support energy needs and enhance the flavor of your meals.

4. **Bone Broth:**

   - Prepare or purchase high-quality bone broth to supplement your diet. Bone broth provides collagen, gelatin, and additional nutrients that can be beneficial for joint health, skin, and overall well-being.

5. **Salt and Seasonings:**

   - Use high-quality salts and seasonings to enhance the taste of your carnivore meals. Opt for unprocessed salts like sea salt or Himalayan salt and experiment with seasonings like black pepper, garlic powder, or herbs to add variety.

Grocery Shopping Guide for Women Over 60:

1. **Selecting Fresh Produce:**

   - While the Carnivore Diet primarily focuses on animal products, consider incorporating fresh herbs and leafy greens for added micronutrients and flavor. Selecting nutrient-dense vegetables can contribute to overall health without compromising the principles of the diet.

2. **Dairy Choices:**

   - Choose high-quality dairy products such as full-fat cheese and cream if tolerated. These can provide additional sources of fat and essential nutrients for women over 60.

3. **Supplements:**

   - Based on individual health needs, consider supplements such as vitamin D, calcium, and magnesium. Consulting with healthcare professionals will help determine the necessity of supplements based on your specific health requirements.

4. **Ethical and Sustainable Meat Sourcing:**

   - When shopping for meat, prioritize ethical and sustainable sourcing. Look for labels indicating grass-fed, pasture-raised, and responsibly sourced options to minimize environmental impact and support humane practices.

5. **Meal Planning:**

- Plan your meals in advance to ensure a balanced and varied carnivore diet. This includes incorporating different cuts of meat, organ meats, and occasionally adding dairy or herbs for flavor and additional nutrients.

CHAPTER 3

CARNIVORE BASICS

The Carnivore Diet is rooted in the exclusive consumption of animal-based foods, emphasizing the importance of high-quality sources to meet nutritional needs. In this Cookbook, we delve into the basics of the Carnivore Diet, exploring different types of animal-based foods, the significance of opting for high-quality meat, and the valuable role of organ meats in providing a nutrient boost.

1. **Types of Animal-Based Foods:**

   - The foundation of the Carnivore Diet is laid with a variety of animal-based foods. These include:

     - **Red Meat:** Beef, lamb, and venison are rich in protein, iron, zinc, and B vitamins.

     - **Poultry:** Chicken and turkey offer lean protein and essential nutrients.

     - **Fish:** Wild-caught fish provides omega-3 fatty acids, protein, and various minerals.

     - **Eggs:** A versatile source of complete protein and essential nutrients.

2. **Importance of High-Quality Meat:**

- Opting for high-quality meat is paramount for the success of the Carnivore Diet. Here's why:

    - **Nutrient Density:** High-quality meats offer a rich array of essential nutrients in their most bioavailable forms.

    - **Reduced Toxins:** Grass-fed beef and pasture-raised poultry often have lower levels of environmental toxins compared to conventionally raised counterparts.

    - **Optimal Fatty Acid Profile:** Grass-fed and pasture-raised meats generally contain a healthier balance of omega-3 to omega-6 fatty acids.

Incorporating Organ Meats for Nutrient Boost:

1. **Nutrient Density of Organ Meats:**

- Organ meats are nutritional powerhouses, packed with essential vitamins and minerals. Examples include liver, heart, kidney, and tongue.

- **Liver:** An excellent source of vitamin A, B12, iron, and copper. It is often considered one of the most nutrient-dense foods.

- **Heart:** Rich in CoQ10, zinc, and selenium, heart meat supports cardiovascular health.

- **Kidney:** Provides essential nutrients such as B vitamins, iron, and selenium.

2. **Balancing Nutrient Intake:**

   - Incorporating a variety of organ meats ensures a balanced nutrient intake. Each organ meat has a unique nutrient profile, contributing to overall health and preventing potential deficiencies.

3. **Overcoming Taste Concerns:**

   - For those new to organ meats, gradual incorporation and creative cooking methods can help overcome taste concerns. Mixing organ meats with ground meat, using flavorful spices, or incorporating them into stews and casseroles can enhance palatability.

4. **Supplementing Essential Nutrients:**

   - While organ meats provide a wealth of nutrients, it's essential to consider individual dietary needs. If necessary, supplementing specific nutrients can help ensure comprehensive nutritional support.

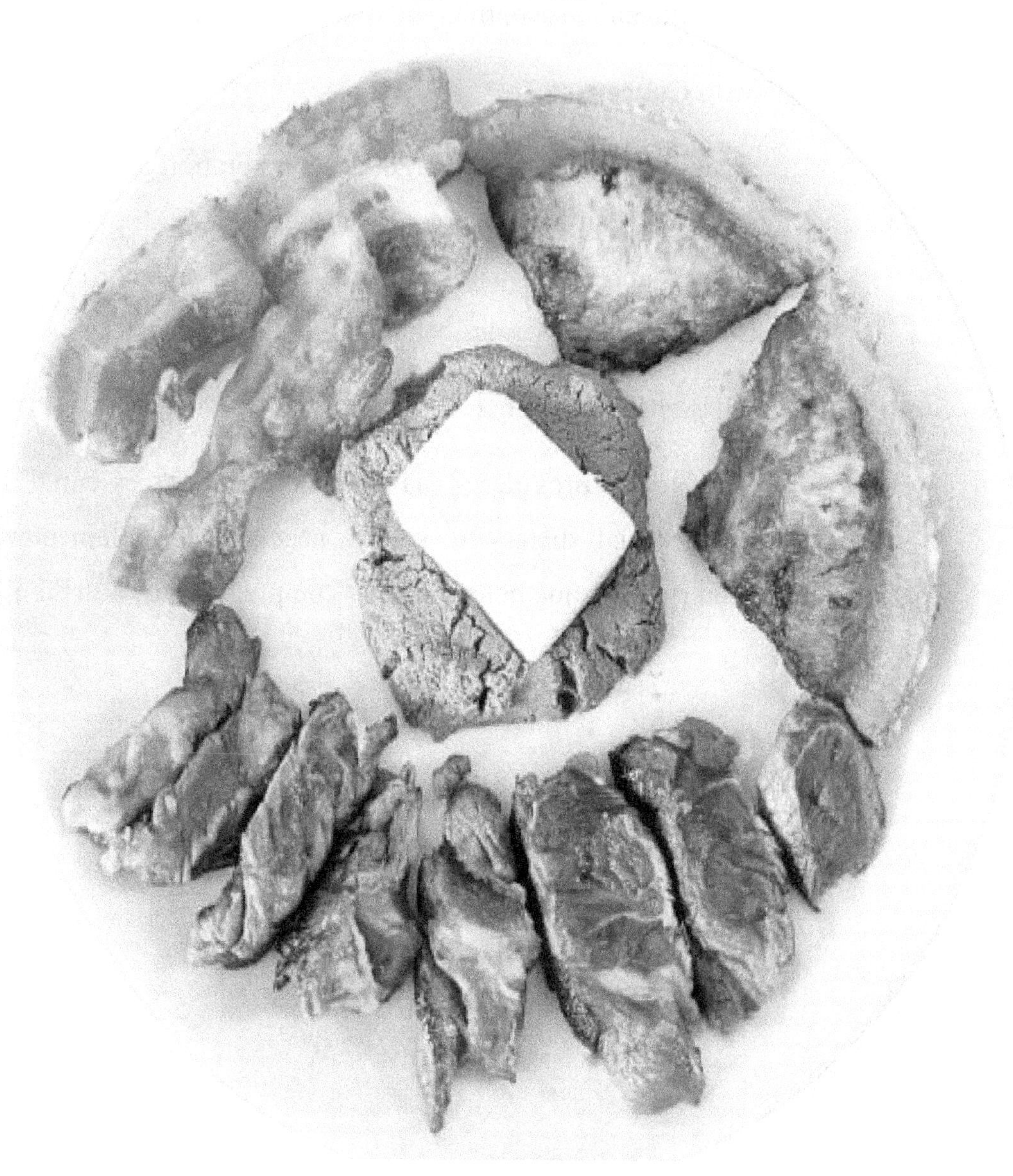

CHAPTER 4

RED MEAT RECIPES

Grilled Ribeye Steak with Herb Butter

Ingredients:

- 2 ribeye steaks (6-8 oz each)

- 2 tbsp olive oil

- Salt and pepper to taste

- 4 tbsp unsalted butter

- 2 cloves minced garlic

- 1 tbsp chopped fresh herbs (rosemary, thyme, or parsley)

Instructions:

1. Preheat the grill to medium-high heat.

2. Rub steaks with olive oil and season with salt and pepper.

3. Grill steaks for 4-6 minutes per side for medium-rare.

4. In a small saucepan, melt butter, add minced garlic and herbs.

5. Pour herb butter over grilled steaks before serving.

Nutritional Information: Approximately 480 calories, 0g carbs, 48g protein, 32g fat, 0g fiber.

Tips: Allow steaks to rest for 5 minutes after grilling to retain juices. Choose grass-fed beef for enhanced nutritional benefits.

Beef and Bacon Skewers

Ingredients:

- 1 lb beef sirloin, cut into cubes

- 8 slices of bacon

- Salt and pepper to taste

- Wooden skewers, soaked in water

Instructions:

1. Preheat the oven to 400°F (200°C).

2. Season beef cubes with salt and pepper.

3. Wrap each beef cube with a slice of bacon and thread onto skewers.

4. Bake for 15-20 minutes or until bacon is crispy.

Nutritional Information: Approximately 350 calories, 0g carbs, 30g protein, 25g

Lamb Chops with Mint Pesto

Cooking Time: 15 minutes **Serving:** 2

Ingredients:

- 4 lamb chops
- Salt and pepper to taste
- 2 tbsp olive oil

Mint Pesto:

- 1 cup fresh mint leaves
- 1/4 cup pine nuts
- 1/4 cup grated Parmesan cheese
- 1 garlic clove
- 1/2 cup extra virgin olive oil

Instructions:

1. Preheat a grill or grill pan to medium-high heat.
2. Season lamb chops with salt and pepper, brush with olive oil.
3. Grill chops for 5-7 minutes per side for medium-rare.
4. For the mint pesto, blend mint, pine nuts, Parmesan, and garlic in a food processor. Gradually add olive oil until smooth.
5. Serve lamb chops drizzled with mint pesto.

Nutritional Information: Approximately 520 calories, 1g carbs, 36g protein, 41g fat, 0g fiber.

Tips: Use the leftover mint pesto as a flavourful topping for other carnivore meals. Adjust garlic and Parmesan quantities to suit personal taste preferences.

Beef Stir-Fry with Vegetables

Cooking Time: 20 minutes **Serving:** 4

Ingredients:

- 1.5 lbs thinly sliced beef (sirloin or flank steak)

- 2 tbsp coconut oil

- 1 broccoli head, cut into florets

- 1 bell pepper, thinly sliced

- Salt and pepper to taste

- 2 tbsp coconut aminos (optional)

Instructions:

1. Heat coconut oil in a skillet over medium-high heat.

2. Add beef slices and cook until browned.

3. Add broccoli and bell pepper, cook until vegetables are tender-crisp.

4. Season with salt and pepper, and add coconut aminos if desired.

5. Serve immediately.

Nutritional Information: Approximately 420 calories, 5g carbs, 40g protein, 27g fat, 2g fiber.

Tips: Experiment with different low-carb vegetables such as asparagus or zucchini. Coconut aminos can add a touch of sweetness to the stir-fry.

Bison Burger Lettuce Wraps

Cooking Time: 15 minutes **Serving:** 3

Ingredients:

- 1 lb ground bison

- Salt and pepper to taste

- 1 tbsp olive oil

- Lettuce leaves (butter or iceberg) for wrapping

Toppings:

- Sliced tomatoes

- Red onion rings

- Mustard or sugar-free ketchup

Instructions:

1. Season bison with salt and pepper, form into burger patties.

2. Heat olive oil in a skillet over medium heat.

3. Cook burgers for 4-5 minutes per side or until desired doneness.

4. Assemble burgers in lettuce wraps, adding toppings of choice.

Nutritional Information: Approximately 360 calories, 1g carbs, 21g protein, 30g fat, 0g fiber.

Tips: Bison is leaner than beef, so be mindful not to overcook to maintain juiciness. Customize toppings to suit personal preferences.

Beef Liver Pâté

Cooking Time: 30 minutes (plus chilling time) **Serving:** 6

Ingredients:

- 1 lb beef liver, sliced

- 1 onion, finely chopped

- 2 cloves garlic, minced

- 1/2 cup unsalted butter

- Salt and pepper to taste

Instructions:

1. Sauté onions and garlic in butter until softened.

2. Add sliced liver, cook for 5-7 minutes.

3. Transfer mixture to a food processor, blend until smooth.

4. Season with salt and pepper, blend again.

5. Chill in the refrigerator for at least 2 hours before serving.

Nutritional Information: Approximately 240 calories, 3g carbs, 18g protein, 18g fat, 0g fiber.

Tips: Spread the pâté on cucumber slices for a low-carb snack. Beef liver is a nutrient powerhouse, rich in vitamins and minerals.

Beef and Egg Breakfast Skillet

Cooking Time: 15 minutes **Serving:** 2

Ingredients:

- 1/2 lb ground beef

- 4 eggs

- Salt and pepper to taste

- Chopped fresh chives for garnish (optional)

Instructions:

1. Brown ground beef in a skillet over medium heat.

2. Create wells in the beef, crack eggs into the wells.

3. Cook until eggs reach desired doneness.

4. Season with salt and pepper, garnish with chives.

Nutritional Information: Approximately 520 calories, 0g carbs, 40g protein, 38g fat, 0g fiber.

Tips: Experiment with spices like cumin or paprika for added flavor. Adjust egg cooking time based on personal preference.

Lamb Stew with Rosemary

Cooking Time: 2 hours **Serving:** 4

Ingredients:

- 2 lbs lamb stew meat, cubed

- 2 tbsp olive oil

- 1 onion, diced

- 2 carrots, sliced

- 2 cloves garlic, minced

- 1 cup beef broth

- 2 sprigs fresh rosemary

- Salt and pepper to taste

Instructions:

1. Heat olive oil in a pot over medium heat.

2. Brown lamb cubes, add onions and garlic.

3. Pour in beef broth, add carrots and rosemary.

4. Simmer on low heat for 1.5-2 hours until lamb is tender.

5. Season with salt and pepper before serving.

Nutritional Information: Approximately 480 calories, 6g carbs, 30g protein, 35g fat, 2g fiber.

Tips: Use bone broth for added richness. Adjust seasoning based on personal taste preferences.

Beef Zoodle Stir-Fry

Cooking Time: 20 minutes **Serving:** 3

Ingredients:

- 1.5 lbs thinly sliced beef (sirloin or flank steak)

- 3 medium zucchinis, spiralized into zoodles

- 2 tbsp coconut oil

- 3 tbsp soy sauce or coconut aminos

- 2 cloves garlic, minced

- Salt and pepper to taste

Instructions:

1. Heat coconut oil in a skillet over medium-high heat.

2. Add beef slices and cook until browned.

3. Add garlic, stir in zoodles and soy sauce.

4. Cook for an additional 5 minutes or until zoodles are tender.

5. Season with salt and pepper before serving.

Nutritional Information: Approximately 400 calories, 7g carbs, 30g protein, 28g fat, 2g fiber.

Tips: Experiment with different low-carb sauces like tamari or fish sauce. Adjust zoodle cooking time based on personal preference.

Beef and Cabbage Rolls

Cooking Time: 45 minutes **Serving:** 3

Ingredients:

- 1 lb ground beef

- 1 head of cabbage

- 1 onion, diced

- 2 cloves garlic, minced

- 1 cup beef broth

- Fresh parsley for garnish

Instructions:

1. Preheat the oven to 375°F (190°C).

2. Boil cabbage leaves until pliable, then drain.

3. Sauté onions and garlic, add ground beef and cook until browned.

4. Place a spoonful of beef mixture on each cabbage leaf, roll up, and secure with toothpicks.

5. Place rolls in a baking dish, pour beef broth over, and bake for 30 minutes.

6. Garnish with fresh parsley before serving.

Nutritional Information: Approximately 320 calories, 10g carbs, 25g protein, 20g fat, 4g fiber.

Tips: Opt for lean ground beef for a lighter option. Remove toothpicks before serving.

CHAPTER 5

PORK RECIPES

Pork Tenderloin with Dijon Mustard Glaze

Cooking Time: 30 minutes **Serving:** 4

Ingredients:

- 1.5 lbs pork tenderloin

- 2 tbsp Dijon mustard

- 1 tbsp olive oil

- 2 cloves garlic, minced

- Fresh parsley for garnish

Instructions:

1. Preheat the oven to 400°F (200°C).
2. Mix Dijon mustard, olive oil, minced garlic, salt, and pepper.
3. Coat pork tenderloin with the mustard mixture.
4. Roast in the oven for 25-30 minutes or until internal temperature reaches 145°F (63°C).
5. Garnish with fresh parsley before serving.

Nutritional Information: Approximately 320 calories, 1g carbs, 40g protein, 17g fat, 0g fiber.

Tips: Let the pork rest for 5 minutes before slicing to retain juices. This glaze also works well on grilled pork.

Pork Belly Crisps

Cooking Time: 2 hours (including baking and cooling) **Serving:** 6

Ingredients:

- 1 lb pork belly, thinly sliced

- Salt and pepper to taste

Instructions:

1. Preheat the oven to 250°F (120°C).

2. Lay pork belly slices on a baking sheet, season with salt and pepper.

3. Bake for 1.5-2 hours or until the slices are crispy.

4. Allow to cool before serving.

Nutritional Information: Approximately 280 calories, 0g carbs, 18g protein, 23g fat, 0g fiber.

Tips: Use a rack on the baking sheet to allow air circulation for extra crispiness. Experiment with seasonings like smoked paprika or garlic powder.

Pork and Cabbage Stir-Fry

Cooking Time: 20 minutes **Serving:** 4

Ingredients:

- 1.5 lbs pork loin, thinly sliced

- 1 small green cabbage, shredded

- 2 tbsp coconut oil

- 2 cloves garlic, minced

- 2 tbsp coconut aminos

- Salt and pepper to taste

Instructions:

1. Heat coconut oil in a wok or skillet over high heat.

2. Add pork slices and cook until browned.

3. Add shredded cabbage and minced garlic, stir-fry until cabbage is tender-crisp.

4. Pour in coconut aminos, season with salt and pepper.

5. Serve hot.

Nutritional Information: Approximately 360 calories, 8g carbs, 30g protein, 23g fat, 4g fiber.

Tips: Adjust coconut aminos to taste preference. Add a dash of sesame oil for extra flavor.

Smoked Paprika Pork Ribs

Cooking Time: 3 hours **Serving:** 4

Ingredients:

- 2 racks of pork ribs
- 2 tbsp smoked paprika
- 1 tbsp garlic powder
- 1 tbsp onion powder
- Salt and pepper to taste

Instructions:

1. Preheat your smoker or grill to 225°F (107°C).
2. Mix smoked paprika, garlic powder, onion powder, salt, and pepper.
3. Rub the spice mixture over the pork ribs.
4. Smoke or grill the ribs for 2.5-3 hours or until tender.

Nutritional Information: Approximately 480 calories, 1g carbs, 32g protein, 38g fat, 0g fiber.

Tips: Use a meat thermometer to ensure ribs reach an internal temperature of 190°F (88°C) for optimal tenderness.

Pork and Mushroom Skillet

Cooking Time: 25 minutes **Serving:** 3

Ingredients:

- 1.5 lbs pork shoulder, cubed
- 1 lb mushrooms, sliced
- 2 tbsp lard or bacon fat
- 1 onion, thinly sliced
- 2 cloves garlic, minced
- Salt and pepper to taste

Instructions:

1. Heat lard or bacon fat in a skillet over medium-high heat.
2. Add pork cubes and brown on all sides.
3. Add sliced mushrooms, onion, and garlic, sauté until mushrooms are tender.
4. Season with salt and pepper.
5. Serve hot.

Nutritional Information: Approximately 420 calories, 6g carbs, 32g protein, 30g fat, 2g fiber.

Tips: Add a splash of bone broth for extra flavor and moisture. Experiment with different mushroom varieties.

Pork Chop Skewers with Herbed Marinade

Cooking Time: 20 minutes **Serving:** 4

Ingredients:

- 4 pork chops, boneless

- 2 tbsp olive oil

- 2 tsp dried thyme

- 1 tsp dried rosemary

- 2 cloves garlic, minced

- Salt and pepper to taste

Instructions:

1. Preheat the grill to medium-high heat.

2. In a bowl, mix olive oil, thyme, rosemary, minced garlic, salt, and pepper.

3. Coat pork chops with the marinade.

4. Thread pork chops onto skewers and grill for 8-10 minutes.

Nutritional Information: Approximately 360 calories, 0g carbs, 30g protein, 25g fat, 0g fiber.

Tips: Marinate the pork chops for at least 30 minutes for optimal flavor. Soak wooden skewers in water to prevent burning.

Pork Loin Roast with Herbs

Cooking Time: 1.5 hours **Serving:** 6

Ingredients:

- 2.5 lbs pork loin roast

- 2 tbsp olive oil

- 2 tsp dried sage

- 1 tsp dried thyme

- 1 tsp dried rosemary

- Salt and pepper to taste

Instructions:

1. Preheat the oven to 375°F (190°C).

2. Rub pork loin with olive oil, sage, thyme, rosemary, salt, and pepper.

3. Roast in the oven for 1-1.5 hours or until the internal temperature reaches 145°F (63°C).

4. Let the roast rest for 10 minutes before slicing.

Nutritional Information: Approximately 250 calories, 0g carbs, 30g protein, 13g fat, 0g fiber.

Tips: Use a meat thermometer to ensure the roast reaches the recommended internal temperature. Serve with pan juices for added flavor.

Pork and Cauliflower Mash Casserole

Cooking Time: 45 minutes **Serving:** 4

Ingredients:

- 1.5 lbs pork shoulder, cubed

- 1 head cauliflower, cut into florets

- 1/2 cup heavy cream

- 1/4 cup butter

- Salt and pepper to taste

Instructions:

1. Preheat the oven to 375°F (190°C).

2. Brown pork cubes in a skillet over medium-high heat.

3. Steam cauliflower until tender, then mash with cream and butter.

4. In a casserole dish, layer pork cubes and cauliflower mash.

5. Bake for 20-25 minutes or until bubbly.

Nutritional Information: Approximately 340 calories, 5g carbs, 30g protein, 22g fat, 2g fiber.

Tips: Experiment with adding cheese on top for a cheesy crust. Adjust the thickness of the cauliflower mash to personal preference.

Pulled Pork Lettuce Wraps

Cooking Time: 6 hours (slow cooker) **Serving:** 6

Ingredients:

- 3 lbs pork shoulder

- 1 cup beef broth

- 1 tbsp smoked paprika

- 1 tbsp garlic powder

- 1 tsp onion powder

- Salt and pepper to taste

- Iceberg lettuce leaves for wrapping

Instructions:

1. Place pork shoulder in a slow cooker, add beef broth.

2. Rub with smoked paprika, garlic powder, onion powder, salt, and pepper.

3. Cook on low for 6 hours or until pork easily shreds.

4. Shred pork and serve in lettuce wraps.

Nutritional Information: Approximately 280 calories, 2g carbs, 28g protein, 18g fat, 1g fiber.

Tips: Top with sugar-free barbecue sauce for added flavor. Use a fork to easily shred the cooked pork.

Pork and Egg Breakfast Skillet

Cooking Time: 20 minutes **Serving:** 3

Ingredients:

- 1 lb ground pork

- 6 eggs

- Salt and pepper to taste

- Chopped fresh chives for garnish (optional)

Instructions:

1. Brown ground pork in a skillet over medium heat.

2. Create wells in the pork, crack eggs into the wells.

3. Cook until eggs reach desired doneness.

4. Season with salt and pepper, garnish with chives.

Nutritional Information: Approximately 520 calories, 0g carbs, 40g protein, 38g fat, 0g fiber.

Tips: Add your favorite spices or herbs for extra flavor. Adjust egg cooking time based on personal preference.

CHAPTER 6

POULTRY RECIPES

Roast Chicken Thighs with Lemon and Herbs

Cooking Time: 45 minutes **Serving:** 4

Ingredients:

- 8 chicken thighs, bone-in, skin-on

- 2 tbsp olive oil

- Zest and juice of 1 lemon

- 2 tsp dried thyme

- Fresh parsley for garnish

Instructions:

1. Preheat the oven to 400°F (200°C).

2. Place chicken thighs in a baking dish, drizzle with olive oil.

3. Season with lemon zest, lemon juice, dried thyme, salt, and pepper.

4. Roast for 40-45 minutes or until chicken reaches an internal temperature of 165°F (74°C).

5. Garnish with fresh parsley before serving.

Nutritional Information: Approximately 400 calories, 0g carbs, 40g protein, 26g fat, 0g fiber.

Tips: For crispy skin, broil for the last 5 minutes. Use a meat thermometer to ensure chicken is fully cooked.

Turkey and Bacon Roll-Ups

Cooking Time: 20 minutes **Serving:** 3

Ingredients:

- 1 lb turkey breast slices

- 6 slices bacon

- Salt and pepper to taste

Instructions:

1. Preheat the oven to 375°F (190°C).

2. Lay turkey slices flat, season with salt and pepper.

3. Roll each turkey slice with a slice of bacon.

4. Place on a baking sheet and bake for 15-20 minutes or until bacon is crispy.

Nutritional Information: Approximately 290 calories, 0g carbs, 35g protein, 16g fat, 0g fiber.

Tips: Secure rolls with toothpicks before baking. Choose uncured bacon for a cleaner option.

Chicken Liver Sauté with Onions

Cooking Time: 15 minutes **Serving:** 2

Ingredients:

- 1 lb chicken livers, cleaned

- 2 tbsp beef tallow or butter

- 1 onion, thinly sliced

- Salt and pepper to taste

Instructions:

1. Heat beef tallow or butter in a skillet over medium heat.

2. Add chicken livers and sliced onions, sauté until livers are no longer pink.

3. Season with salt and pepper.

4. Serve hot.

Nutritional Information: Approximately 320 calories, 3g carbs, 30g protein, 20g fat, 1g fiber.

Tips: Do not overcook the livers to maintain tenderness. Add a splash of red wine for extra flavor.

Grilled Duck Breast with Rosemary

Cooking Time: 20 minutes **Serving:** 2

Ingredients:

- 2 duck breasts, skin-on

- 2 tbsp olive oil

- Fresh rosemary sprigs

- Salt and pepper to taste

Instructions:

1. Preheat the grill to medium-high heat.

2. Score the duck breast skin, rub with olive oil, salt, and pepper.

3. Place duck breasts on the grill, skin side down, and add fresh rosemary.

4. Grill for 8-10 minutes per side or until internal temperature reaches 145°F (63°C).

5. Allow to rest for 5 minutes before slicing.

Nutritional Information: Approximately 480 calories, 0g carbs, 30g protein, 40g fat, 0g fiber.

Tips: Duck breast can be rich, so a little goes a long way. Save the rendered fat for cooking vegetables.

Chicken and Bacon Skewers

Cooking Time: 20 minutes **Serving:** 4

Ingredients:

- 1.5 lbs chicken breast, cut into cubes

- 8 slices bacon

- Salt and pepper to taste

Instructions:

1. Preheat the oven to 400°F (200°C).

2. Season chicken cubes with salt and pepper.

3. Wrap each chicken cube with a slice of bacon and thread onto skewers.

4. Bake for 15-20 minutes or until bacon is crispy.

Nutritional Information: Approximately 350 calories, 0g carbs, 30g protein, 25g fat, 0g fiber.

Tips: Marinate chicken in your favorite spices for added flavor. Soak wooden skewers in water to prevent burning.

Quail Eggs with Butter and Sea Salt

Cooking Time: 5 minutes **Serving:** 2

Ingredients:

- 12 quail eggs

- 2 tbsp butter

- Sea salt to taste

Instructions:

1. Bring a pot of water to a boil and gently add quail eggs.

2. Boil for 4 minutes, then transfer eggs to an ice bath to cool.

3. Peel the eggs and cut in half.

4. Melt butter in a pan, add quail eggs, and sauté for 1 minute.

5. Sprinkle with sea salt before serving.

Nutritional Information: Approximately 240 calories, 0g carbs, 14g protein, 20g fat, 0g fiber.

Tips: Quail eggs are small, so adjust serving size accordingly. These make a delightful and elegant appetizer.

Chicken Thighs with Garlic and Lemon

Cooking Time: 35 minutes **Serving:** 4

Ingredients:

- 8 chicken thighs, bone-in, skin-on

- 4 cloves garlic, minced

- Zest and juice of 1 lemon

- 2 tbsp olive oil

- Salt and pepper to taste

Instructions:

1. Preheat the oven to 375°F (190°C).

2. Mix minced garlic, lemon zest, lemon juice, and olive oil.

3. Coat chicken thighs with the mixture, season with salt and pepper.

4. Roast for 30-35 minutes or until chicken reaches an internal temperature of 165°F (74°C).

Nutritional Information: Approximately 380 calories, 1g carbs, 40g protein, 24g fat, 0g fiber.

Tips: For extra flavor, let the chicken marinate in the mixture for 30 minutes before roasting. Use fresh herbs for added aroma.

Turkey Burger Lettuce Wraps

Cooking Time: 15 minutes **Serving:** 3

Ingredients:

- 1 lb ground turkey

- Salt and pepper to taste

- 1 tbsp olive oil

- Lettuce leaves (butter or iceberg) for wrapping

Toppings:

- Sliced tomatoes

- Red onion rings

- Mustard or sugar-free ketchup

Instructions:

1. Season ground turkey with salt and pepper, form into burger patties.

2. Heat olive oil in a skillet over medium heat.

3. Cook burgers for 4-5 minutes per side or until cooked through.

4. Assemble burgers in lettuce wraps, adding toppings of choice.

Nutritional Information: Approximately 330 calories, 0g carbs, 30g protein, 22g fat, 0g fiber.

Tips: Customize toppings to suit personal preferences. Turkey is lean, so avoid overcooking to retain moisture.

Chicken Liver Pâté with Bacon

Cooking Time: 30 minutes (plus chilling time) **Serving:** 6

Ingredients:

- 1 lb chicken livers

- 8 slices bacon, cooked and crumbled

- 1/2 cup unsalted butter

- 2 cloves garlic, minced

- Salt and pepper to taste

Instructions:

1. Sauté chicken livers and minced garlic in butter until no longer pink.

2. Transfer mixture to a food processor, blend until smooth.

3. Stir in crumbled bacon, season with salt and pepper.

4. Chill in the refrigerator for at least 2 hours before serving.

Nutritional Information: Approximately 280 calories, 2g carbs, 20g protein, 22g fat, 0g fiber.

Tips: Spread the pâté on cucumber slices for a low-carb snack. Adjust garlic and seasoning quantities based on taste preference.

Lemon Herb Turkey Wings

Cooking Time: 1.5 hours **Serving:** 4

Ingredients:

- 2 lbs turkey wings
- Zest and juice of 1 lemon
- 2 tbsp olive oil
- 2 tsp dried rosemary
- 1 tsp dried thyme
- Salt and pepper to taste

Instructions:

1. Preheat the oven to 375°F (190°C).
2. Mix lemon zest, lemon juice, olive oil, rosemary, thyme, salt, and pepper.
3. Coat turkey wings with the mixture.
4. Roast in the oven for 1-1.5 hours or until wings reach an internal temperature of 165°F (74°C).

Nutritional Information: Approximately 300 calories, 0g carbs, 30g protein, 20g fat, 0g fiber.

Tips: Baste the wings with the lemon herb mixture every 30 minutes for enhanced flavor. Use a meat thermometer to ensure proper cooking.

CHAPTER 7

SEAFOOD RECIPES

Garlic Butter Shrimp Skewers

Cooking Time: 15 minutes **Serving:** 3

Ingredients:

- 1 lb large shrimp, peeled and deveined

- 4 tbsp unsalted butter, melted

- 4 cloves garlic, minced

- Salt and pepper to taste

Instructions:

1. Preheat the grill to medium-high heat.

2. In a bowl, toss shrimp with melted butter, minced garlic, salt, and pepper.

3. Thread shrimp onto skewers and grill for 2-3 minutes per side or until opaque.

4. Serve hot.

Nutritional Information: Approximately 280 calories, 0g carbs, 24g protein, 20g fat, 0g fiber.

Tips: Use fresh shrimp for optimal flavor. Soak wooden skewers in water to prevent burning.

Seared Scallops with Lemon and Herb Butter

Cooking Time: 10 minutes **Serving:** 2

Ingredients:

- 1 lb sea scallops

- 2 tbsp clarified butter

- Zest and juice of 1 lemon

- 1 tsp chopped fresh parsley

- Salt and pepper to taste

Instructions:

1. Pat scallops dry and season with salt and pepper.

2. Heat clarified butter in a skillet over medium-high heat.

3. Sear scallops for 2-3 minutes per side until golden brown.

4. Sprinkle with lemon zest, lemon juice, and chopped parsley before serving.

Nutritional Information: Approximately 240 calories, 3g carbs, 20g protein, 16g fat, 0g fiber.

Tips: Ensure scallops are dry before cooking for a perfect sear. Use a non-stick skillet for easier cooking.

Grilled Salmon Steaks with Dill

Cooking Time: 15 minutes **Serving:** 2

Ingredients:

- 2 salmon steaks

- 2 tbsp olive oil

- 1 tbsp fresh dill, chopped

- Salt and pepper to taste

- Lemon wedges for serving

Instructions:

1. Preheat the grill to medium-high heat.

2. Brush salmon steaks with olive oil, sprinkle with chopped dill, salt, and pepper.

3. Grill for 6-8 minutes per side or until fish flakes easily.

4. Serve with lemon wedges.

Nutritional Information: Approximately 400 calories, 0g carbs, 40g protein, 26g fat, 0g fiber.

Tips: Choose wild-caught salmon for optimal omega-3 fatty acids. Grilling enhances the natural flavors of the fish.

Butter-Basted Lobster Tails

Cooking Time: 20 minutes **Serving:** 2

Ingredients:

- 2 lobster tails, split in half

- 4 tbsp unsalted butter, melted

- 2 cloves garlic, minced

- Salt and pepper to taste

Instructions:

1. Preheat the broiler in your oven.

2. Place lobster tails on a baking sheet, shell side down.

3. Mix melted butter, minced garlic, salt, and pepper.

4. Brush lobster tails with the butter mixture and broil for 10-12 minutes.

5. Serve hot.

Nutritional Information: Approximately 320 calories, 0g carbs, 28g protein, 22g fat, 0g fiber.

Tips: Keep an eye on the lobster tails to prevent overcooking. Basting with butter enhances flavor and keeps the meat moist.

Tuna Steak with Lemon and Rosemary

Cooking Time: 10 minutes **Serving:** 2

Ingredients:

- 2 tuna steaks

- 2 tbsp olive oil

- Zest and juice of 1 lemon

- 1 tsp dried rosemary

- Salt and pepper to taste

Instructions:

1. Preheat a skillet or grill pan over medium-high heat.

2. Brush tuna steaks with olive oil, sprinkle with lemon zest, lemon juice, rosemary, salt, and pepper.

3. Cook for 3-4 minutes per side or until desired doneness.

4. Serve hot.

Nutritional Information: Approximately 300 calories, 0g carbs, 40g protein, 16g fat, 0g fiber.

Tips: Searing tuna quickly on high heat preserves its tenderness. Adjust cooking time based on personal preference.

Sardine Salad with Olive Oil and Lemon

Preparation Time: 10 minutes **Serving:** 1

Ingredients:

- 1 can sardines in olive oil

- Mixed salad greens

- 1 tbsp olive oil

- Zest and juice of 1 lemon

- Salt and pepper to taste

Instructions:

1. Arrange mixed salad greens on a plate.

2. Open the can of sardines and place them on top of the greens.

3. Drizzle with olive oil, sprinkle with lemon zest, lemon juice, salt, and pepper.

4. Toss lightly before serving.

Nutritional Information: Approximately 320 calories, 2g carbs, 20g protein, 26g fat, 1g fiber.

Tips: Sardines are rich in omega-3 fatty acids and calcium. Choose sardines packed in olive oil for added flavor.

Shrimp and Avocado Salad

Preparation Time: 15 minutes **Serving:** 2

Ingredients:

- 1 lb shrimp, peeled and deveined

- 2 avocados, diced

- 1/4 cup olive oil

- Zest and juice of 1 lime

- Salt and pepper to taste

- Fresh cilantro for garnish

Instructions:

1. Cook shrimp in a skillet over medium-high heat until pink.

2. In a bowl, combine diced avocados, olive oil, lime zest, lime juice, salt, and pepper.

3. Add cooked shrimp to the bowl and toss.

4. Garnish with fresh cilantro before serving.

Nutritional Information: Approximately 420 calories, 8g carbs, 30g protein, 32g fat, 6g fiber.

Tips: Opt for large shrimp for a satisfying bite. Lime adds a refreshing citrusy twist to the salad.

Anchovy and Bacon Wrapped Asparagus

Cooking Time: 15 minutes **Serving:** 2

Ingredients:

- 1 bunch asparagus spears
- 8 anchovy fillets
- 4 slices bacon
- Olive oil for drizzling
- Salt and pepper to taste

Instructions:

1. Preheat the oven to 400°F (200°C).
2. Wrap each asparagus spear with an anchovy fillet, then with a slice of bacon.
3. Place on a baking sheet, drizzle with olive oil, and season with salt and pepper.
4. Bake for 10-12 minutes or until bacon is crispy.
5. Serve warm.

Nutritional Information: Approximately 280 calories, 4g carbs, 18g protein, 22g fat, 2g fiber.

Tips: Anchovies provide a savory kick while bacon adds a smoky flavor. Adjust baking time based on personal preference.

Canned Tuna and Egg Salad

Preparation Time: 10 minutes **Serving:** 2

Ingredients:

- 2 cans tuna in water, drained

- 4 hard-boiled eggs, chopped

- 1/4 cup mayonnaise

- 1 tbsp Dijon mustard

- Salt and pepper to taste

Instructions:

1. In a bowl, combine drained tuna, chopped hard-boiled eggs, mayonnaise, and Dijon mustard.

2. Mix well and season with salt and pepper.

3. Serve chilled.

Nutritional Information: Approximately 450 calories, 2g carbs, 50g protein, 26g fat, 0g fiber.

Tips: Use a good-quality mayonnaise for the best flavor. Serve over lettuce leaves or cucumber slices.

Broiled Mackerel with Lemon and Garlic

Cooking Time: 15 minutes **Serving:** 2

Ingredients:

- 2 mackerel fillets

- 2 tbsp olive oil

- Zest and juice of 1 lemon

- 2 cloves garlic, minced

- Salt and pepper to taste

Instructions:

1. Preheat the broiler in your oven.

2. Place mackerel fillets on a baking sheet.

3. Mix olive oil, lemon zest, lemon juice, minced garlic, salt, and pepper.

4. Brush the mixture over the mackerel and broil for 6-8 minutes or until fish flakes easily.

5. Serve hot.

Nutritional Information: Approximately 340 calories, 0g carbs, 30g protein, 24g fat, 0g fiber.

Tips: Mackerel is a fatty fish rich in omega-3s. Adjust the amount of garlic based on personal preference.

CHAPTER 8

NOSE TO TAIL RECIPES

Beef Heart Skewers with Herb Marinade

Cooking Time: 20 minutes **Serving:** 4

Ingredients:

- 1 beef heart, cleaned and cubed

- 4 tbsp olive oil

- 2 tsp dried oregano

- 1 tsp dried thyme

Instructions:

1. Preheat the grill to medium-high heat.

2. In a bowl, mix olive oil, dried oregano, dried thyme, salt, and pepper.

3. Coat beef heart cubes with the marinade and thread onto skewers.

4. Grill for 8-10 minutes, turning occasionally, until cooked to desired doneness.

5. Serve hot.

Nutritional Information: Approximately 280 calories, 0g carbs, 36g protein, 14g fat, 0g fiber.

Tips: Marinate the beef heart for at least 30 minutes for enhanced flavor. Use a meat thermometer to avoid overcooking.

Liver Pâté with Bacon

Cooking Time: 30 minutes (plus chilling time) **Serving:** 6

Ingredients:

- 1 lb beef liver

- 8 slices bacon, cooked and crumbled

- 1/2 cup unsalted butter

- 2 cloves garlic, minced

- Salt and pepper to taste

Instructions:

1. Sauté beef liver and minced garlic in butter until no longer pink.

2. Transfer the mixture to a food processor, blend until smooth.

3. Stir in crumbled bacon, season with salt and pepper.

4. Chill in the refrigerator for at least 2 hours before serving.

Nutritional Information: Approximately 280 calories, 2g carbs, 20g protein, 22g fat, 0g fiber.

Tips: Spread the pâté on cucumber slices for a low-carb snack. Adjust garlic and seasoning quantities based on taste preference.

Braised Ox Tongue with Red Wine

Cooking Time: 3 hours **Serving:** 4

Ingredients:

- 1 ox tongue

- 2 cups red wine

- 1 onion, sliced

- 2 cloves garlic, minced

- 2 tbsp lard or tallow

- Salt and pepper to taste

Instructions:

1. Preheat the oven to 300°F (150°C).

2. In a Dutch oven, heat lard or tallow over medium-high heat.

3. Sear the ox tongue until browned on all sides.

4. Add red wine, onion, garlic, salt, and pepper.

5. Cover and braise in the oven for 2.5-3 hours or until tender.

6. Slice and serve.

Nutritional Information: Approximately 340 calories, 2g carbs, 30g protein, 22g fat, 0g fiber.

Tips: Braising the ox tongue in red wine adds depth to the flavor. Serve with cauliflower mash or roasted vegetables.

Pork Kidney Stir-Fry with Herbs

Cooking Time: 15 minutes **Serving:** 2

Ingredients:

- 2 pork kidneys, cleaned and sliced

- 2 tbsp beef tallow or lard

- 1 tsp dried rosemary

- 1 tsp dried thyme

- Salt and pepper to taste

Instructions:

1. Heat beef tallow or lard in a skillet over medium-high heat.

2. Add sliced pork kidneys and stir-fry until no longer pink.

3. Season with dried rosemary, dried thyme, salt, and pepper.

4. Cook for an additional 5 minutes, ensuring kidneys are fully cooked.

5. Serve hot.

Nutritional Information: Approximately 260 calories, 0g carbs, 28g protein, 16g fat, 0g fiber.

Tips: Soaking pork kidneys in milk for a few hours before cooking can help reduce any potential strong flavor.

Lamb Brain Fritters

Cooking Time: 20 minutes **Serving:** 3

Ingredients:

- 3 lamb brains

- 2 eggs

- 1/2 cup almond flour

- 2 tbsp ghee or tallow

- Salt and pepper to taste

Instructions:

1. In a bowl, whisk eggs and season with salt and pepper.

2. Dredge lamb brains in almond flour, then dip in the beaten eggs.

3. Heat ghee or tallow in a skillet over medium heat.

4. Fry lamb brains for 3-4 minutes per side or until golden brown.

5. Serve hot.

Nutritional Information: Approximately 330 calories, 2g carbs, 20g protein, 26g fat, 1g fiber.

Tips: Almond flour adds a crispy coating to the lamb brains. Use fresh brains for the best texture.

Roasted Bone Marrow with Herb Butter

Cooking Time: 25 minutes **Serving:** 2

Ingredients:

- 4 beef marrow bones, halved lengthwise

- 4 tbsp unsalted butter, softened

- 2 tsp chopped fresh parsley

- Salt and pepper to taste

Instructions:

1. Preheat the oven to 450°F (230°C).

2. Place marrow bones on a baking sheet, cut side up.

3. Roast for 20 minutes or until the marrow is easily scoopable.

4. Mix softened butter with chopped fresh parsley, salt, and pepper.

5. Spread the herb butter over the roasted marrow and serve.

Nutritional Information: Approximately 400 calories, 0g carbs, 10g protein, 40g fat, 0g fiber.

Tips: Serve with a side of coarse salt and thinly sliced radishes for a refreshing contrast.

Beef Spleen Sauté with Onions

Cooking Time: 20 minutes **Serving:** 2

Ingredients:

- 1 beef spleen, cleaned and sliced

- 1 onion, thinly sliced

- 2 tbsp beef tallow or lard

- 2 cloves garlic, minced

- Salt and pepper to taste

Instructions:

1. Heat beef tallow or lard in a skillet over medium-high heat.

2. Add sliced beef spleen and sauté until browned.

3. Add thinly sliced onion and minced garlic, continue to sauté until onion is tender.

4. Season with salt and pepper.

5. Serve hot.

Nutritional Information: Approximately 280 calories, 2g carbs, 30g protein, 18g fat, 1g fiber.

Tips: Quick cooking maintains the tenderness of beef spleen. Pair with a side of sautéed greens.

Tripe Stew with Tomato and Spices

Cooking Time: 2 hours **Serving:** 4

Ingredients:

- 1 lb beef tripe, cleaned and sliced

- 1 can diced tomatoes

- 1 onion, chopped

- 2 cloves garlic, minced

- 2 tsp ground cumin

- 1 tsp smoked paprika

- Salt and pepper to taste

Instructions:

1. In a pot, combine beef tripe, diced tomatoes, chopped onion, minced garlic, ground cumin, smoked paprika, salt, and pepper.

2. Bring to a simmer, then reduce heat and let it simmer for 2 hours.

3. Adjust seasoning and serve hot.

Nutritional Information: Approximately 320 calories, 8g carbs, 30g protein, 18g fat, 2g fiber.

Tips: Serve the tripe stew over cauliflower rice for a complete meal. Cooking longer enhances the tenderness of the tripe.

Lamb Testicles with Lemon and Garlic

Cooking Time: 15 minutes **Serving:** 2

Ingredients:

- 4 lamb testicles, cleaned

- 2 tbsp olive oil

- Zest and juice of 1 lemon

- 3 cloves garlic, minced

- Salt and pepper to taste

Instructions:

1. Preheat a skillet over medium-high heat.

2. Mix olive oil, lemon zest, lemon juice, minced garlic, salt, and pepper.

3. Sauté lamb testicles for 5-7 minutes or until cooked through.

4. Pour the lemon-garlic mixture over the testicles before serving.

Nutritional Information: Approximately 260 calories, 2g carbs, 30g protein, 14g fat, 0g fiber.

Tips: Choose fresh lamb testicles for the best flavor. Searing quickly maintains their tenderness.

Pork Tail Stew with Rosemary

Cooking Time: 2 hours **Serving:** 4

Ingredients:

- 2 lbs pork tails

- 1 onion, chopped

- 2 carrots, sliced

- 2 sprigs fresh rosemary

- 4 cups beef or bone broth

- Salt and pepper to taste

Instructions:

1. In a pot, combine pork tails, chopped onion, sliced carrots, fresh rosemary, beef or bone broth, salt, and pepper.

2. Bring to a boil, then reduce heat and let it simmer for 2 hours.

3. Discard rosemary sprigs before serving.

Nutritional Information: Approximately 400 calories, 4g carbs, 30g protein, 30g fat, 1g fiber.

Tips: Slow cooking the pork tails enhances the flavor and tenderness. Serve the stew with a side of roasted vegetables.

CHAPTER 9
28 DAY MEAL PLAN

Day 1:

- **Breakfast:** Quail Eggs with Butter and Sea Salt

- **Lunch:** Turkey and Bacon Roll-Ups

- **Dinner:** Beef Heart Skewers with Herb Marinade

- **Snack:** Chicken Liver Pâté with Bacon

Day 2:

- **Breakfast:** Roasted Bone Marrow with Herb Butter

- **Lunch:** Seared Scallops with Lemon and Herb Butter

- **Dinner:** Braised Ox Tongue with Red Wine

- **Snack:** Anchovy and Bacon Wrapped Asparagus

Day 3:

- **Breakfast:** Grilled Duck Breast with Rosemary

- **Lunch:** Tuna Steak with Lemon and Rosemary

- **Dinner:** Liver Pâté with Bacon

- **Snack:** Quail Eggs with Butter and Sea Salt

Day 4:

- **Breakfast:** Chicken Thighs with Garlic and Lemon

- **Lunch:** Turkey Burger Lettuce Wraps

- **Dinner:** Pork Kidney Stir-Fry with Herbs

- **Snack:** Butter-Basted Lobster Tails

Day 5:

- **Breakfast:** Chicken Liver Sauté with Onions

- **Lunch:** Chicken and Bacon Skewers

- **Dinner:** Grilled Salmon Steaks with Dill

- **Snack:** Sardine Salad with Olive Oil and Lemon

Day 6:

- **Breakfast:** Lemon Herb Turkey Wings

- **Lunch:** Shrimp and Avocado Salad

- **Dinner:** Lamb Brain Fritters

- **Snack:** Beef Heart Skewers with Herb Marinade

Day 7:

- **Breakfast:** Grilled Duck Breast with Rosemary

- **Lunch:** Chicken Liver Pâté with Bacon

- **Dinner:** Braised Ox Tongue with Red Wine

- **Snack:** Anchovy and Bacon Wrapped Asparagus

Day 8:

- **Breakfast:** Roasted Bone Marrow with Herb Butter

- **Lunch:** Seared Scallops with Lemon and Herb Butter

- **Dinner:** Liver Pâté with Bacon

- **Snack:** Quail Eggs with Butter and Sea Salt

Day 9:

- **Breakfast:** Chicken Thighs with Garlic and Lemon

- **Lunch:** Turkey Burger Lettuce Wraps

- **Dinner:** Pork Kidney Stir-Fry with Herbs

- **Snack:** Butter-Basted Lobster Tails

Day 10:

- **Breakfast:** Chicken Liver Sauté with Onions

- **Lunch:** Chicken and Bacon Skewers

- **Dinner:** Grilled Salmon Steaks with Dill

- **Snack:** Sardine Salad with Olive Oil and Lemon

Day 11:

- **Breakfast:** Lemon Herb Turkey Wings

- **Lunch:** Shrimp and Avocado Salad

- **Dinner:** Lamb Brain Fritters

- **Snack:** Beef Heart Skewers with Herb Marinade

Day 12:

- **Breakfast:** Grilled Duck Breast with Rosemary

- **Lunch:** Chicken Liver Pâté with Bacon

- **Dinner:** Braised Ox Tongue with Red Wine

- **Snack:** Anchovy and Bacon Wrapped Asparagus

Day 13:

- **Breakfast:** Roasted Bone Marrow with Herb Butter

- **Lunch:** Seared Scallops with Lemon and Herb Butter

- **Dinner:** Liver Pâté with Bacon

- **Snack:** Quail Eggs with Butter and Sea Salt

Day 14:

- **Breakfast:** Chicken Thighs with Garlic and Lemon

- **Lunch:** Turkey Burger Lettuce Wraps

- **Dinner:** Pork Kidney Stir-Fry with Herbs

- **Snack:** Butter-Basted Lobster Tails

Day 15:

- **Breakfast:** Chicken Liver Sauté with Onions

- **Lunch:** Chicken and Bacon Skewers

- **Dinner:** Grilled Salmon Steaks with Dill

- **Snack:** Sardine Salad with Olive Oil and Lemon

Day 16:

- **Breakfast:** Lemon Herb Turkey Wings

- **Lunch:** Shrimp and Avocado Salad

- **Dinner:** Lamb Brain Fritters

- **Snack:** Beef Heart Skewers with Herb Marinade

Day 17:

- **Breakfast:** Grilled Duck Breast with Rosemary

- **Lunch:** Chicken Liver Pâté with Bacon

- **Dinner:** Braised Ox Tongue with Red Wine

- **Snack:** Anchovy and Bacon Wrapped Asparagus

Day 18:

- **Breakfast:** Roasted Bone Marrow with Herb Butter

- **Lunch:** Seared Scallops with Lemon and Herb Butter

- **Dinner:** Liver Pâté with Bacon

- **Snack:** Quail Eggs with Butter and Sea Salt

Day 19:

- **Breakfast:** Chicken Thighs with Garlic and Lemon

- **Lunch:** Turkey Burger Lettuce Wraps

- **Dinner:** Pork Kidney Stir-Fry with Herbs

- **Snack:** Butter-Basted Lobster Tails

Day 20:

- **Breakfast:** Chicken Liver Sauté with Onions

- **Lunch:** Chicken and Bacon Skewers

- **Dinner:** Grilled Salmon Steaks with Dill

- **Snack:** Sardine Salad with Olive Oil and Lemon

Day 21:

- **Breakfast:** Lemon Herb Turkey Wings

- **Lunch:** Shrimp and Avocado Salad

- **Dinner:** Lamb Brain Fritters

- **Snack:** Beef Heart Skewers with Herb Marinade

Day 22:

- **Breakfast:** Grilled Duck Breast with Rosemary

- **Lunch:** Chicken Liver Pâté with Bacon

- **Dinner:** Braised Ox Tongue with Red Wine

- **Snack:** Anchovy and Bacon Wrapped Asparagus

Day 23:

- **Breakfast:** Roasted Bone Marrow with Herb Butter

- **Lunch:** Seared Scallops with Lemon and Herb Butter

- **Dinner:** Liver Pâté with Bacon

- **Snack:** Quail Eggs with Butter and Sea Salt

Day 24:

- **Breakfast:** Chicken Thighs with Garlic and Lemon

- **Lunch:** Turkey Burger Lettuce Wraps

- **Dinner:** Pork Kidney Stir-Fry with Herbs

- **Snack:** Butter-Basted Lobster Tails

Day 25:

- **Breakfast:** Chicken Liver Sauté with Onions

- **Lunch:** Chicken and Bacon Skewers

- **Dinner:** Grilled Salmon Steaks with Dill

- **Snack:** Sardine Salad with Olive Oil and Lemon

Day 26:

- **Breakfast:** Lemon Herb Turkey Wings

- **Lunch:** Shrimp and Avocado Salad

- **Dinner:** Lamb Brain Fritters

- **Snack:** Beef Heart Skewers with Herb Marinade

Day 27:

- **Breakfast:** Grilled Duck Breast with Rosemary

- **Lunch:** Chicken Liver Pâté with Bacon

- **Dinner:** Braised Ox Tongue with Red Wine

- **Snack:** Anchovy and Bacon Wrapped Asparagus

Day 28:

- **Breakfast:** Roasted Bone Marrow with Herb Butter

- **Lunch:** Seared Scallops with Lemon and Herb Butter

- **Dinner:** Liver Pâté with Bacon

- **Snack:** Quail Eggs with Butter and Sea Salt

CONCLUSION

In concluding this carnivore culinary adventure, my dear readers, I want to express my heartfelt gratitude for joining me on this journey. We've explored the rich and flavorful world of carnivore recipes, embracing a lifestyle that not only nourishes our bodies but ignites a passion for wholesome, satisfying meals.

As you close the pages of this cookbook, I encourage you to reflect on the changes you've witnessed – not just in your approach to food but in your overall well-being. The carnivore diet is more than a way of eating; it's a philosophy that celebrates the simplicity of nature's bounty, providing us with the tools to reclaim our health and vitality.

I am eager to hear about your experiences, your kitchen triumphs, and the moments of culinary joy these recipes have brought into your life. Your feedback is a crucial ingredient in this ongoing culinary experiment, and I invite you to share your thoughts, insights, and any personal adaptations you've made to the recipes.

Did a particular dish become a household favorite? Were there challenges or triumphs you encountered along the way? Your honest reviews can serve as a guide for others embarking on this carnivore journey, helping to create a community of like-minded individuals committed to their health and culinary exploration.

Feel free to reach out through social media, email, or any other platform where we can connect. Your stories inspire me, and I am genuinely excited to continue this dialogue, sharing in the collective wisdom of a community committed to vibrant living through mindful eating.

As you savor the last bites of your carnivore-inspired creations, I leave you with this thought: The journey to a healthier, happier you is ongoing, and the kitchen is your canvas. Keep experimenting, keep relishing the flavors, and most importantly, enjoy every moment of this culinary adventure.

Thank you for being a part of this carnivore community. Your presence has made this journey all the more enriching. Until we meet again in the world of delicious possibilities, happy cooking, and bon appétit!

BONUS CHAPTER

10 DESSERTS RECIPES

1. Bacon-Wrapped Dates

Cooking Time: 15 minutes **Serving:** 4

Ingredients:

- 8 Medjool dates, pitted

- 4 slices bacon, cut in half

Instructions:

1. Preheat the oven to 375°F (190°C).

2. Wrap each date with half a slice of bacon.

3. Place on a baking sheet and bake for 12-15 minutes or until bacon is crispy.

4. Allow to cool slightly before serving.

Nutritional Information: Approximately 180 calories, 20g protein, 12g fat, 12g carbs, 2g fiber.

Tips: Choose thick-cut bacon for a satisfying crunch. Ensure dates are pitted before wrapping.

2. Beef Tallow Chocolate Truffles

Preparation Time: 20 minutes (plus chilling time) **Serving:** 6

Ingredients:

- 1 cup beef tallow, melted

- 1 cup unsweetened cocoa powder

- 1/4 cup powdered erythritol (optional)

- Pinch of salt

Instructions:

1. Mix melted beef tallow, cocoa powder, powdered erythritol, and a pinch of salt until well combined.

2. Form small truffle balls and place them on a parchment-lined tray.

3. Chill in the refrigerator for at least 2 hours before serving.

Nutritional Information: Approximately 200 calories, 4g protein, 20g fat, 5g carbs, 3g fiber.

Tips: Adjust sweetness by adding more or less erythritol. Roll truffles in cocoa powder or crushed nuts for variation.

3. Coconut Oil Cinnamon Fat Bombs

Preparation Time: 15 minutes (plus freezing time) **Serving:** 8

Ingredients:

- 1 cup coconut oil, melted

- 1 teaspoon ground cinnamon

- Stevia or monk fruit sweetener to taste

Instructions:

1. Mix melted coconut oil with ground cinnamon and sweetener.

2. Pour the mixture into silicone molds or ice cube trays.

3. Freeze until solid, then pop out and serve.

Nutritional Information: Approximately 130 calories, 0g protein, 14g fat, 0g carbs, 0g fiber.

Tips: Experiment with different spices like nutmeg or cardamom for flavor variations.

4. Pork Rind "Cereal" with Berries

Preparation Time: 5 minutes **Serving:** 1

Ingredients:

- 1 cup crushed pork rinds

- 1/2 cup heavy cream

- 1/2 cup mixed berries (strawberries, blueberries)

Instructions:

1. Mix crushed pork rinds with heavy cream in a bowl.

2. Top with mixed berries and enjoy.

Nutritional Information: Approximately 400 calories, 15g protein, 35g fat, 5g carbs, 2g fiber.

Tips: Add a dollop of whipped cream or a sprinkle of cinnamon for extra indulgence.

5. Bone Marrow Custard

Cooking Time: 30 minutes (plus chilling time) **Serving:** 4

Ingredients:

- 2 cups bone marrow, cooked and mashed

- 1 cup heavy cream

- 1/4 cup powdered erythritol

- 1 teaspoon vanilla extract

Instructions:

1. In a bowl, mix mashed bone marrow with heavy cream, erythritol, and vanilla extract.

2. Blend until smooth and pour into serving dishes.

3. Chill in the refrigerator for at least 4 hours before serving.

Nutritional Information: Approximately 300 calories, 5g protein, 28g fat, 4g carbs, 0g fiber.

Tips: Garnish with a sprinkle of nutmeg or a few berries before serving.

6. Chicken Liver Pâté Stuffed Avocado

Preparation Time: 15 minutes **Serving:** 2

Ingredients:

- 1/2 cup chicken liver pâté

- 1 ripe avocado, halved and pitted

Instructions:

1. Fill each avocado half with a generous spoonful of chicken liver pâté.

2. Serve immediately.

Nutritional Information: Approximately 400 calories, 15g protein, 35g fat, 8g carbs, 6g fiber.

Tips: Choose a smooth and creamy chicken liver pâté for the best texture.

7. Salmon and Cream Cheese Roll-Ups

Preparation Time: 10 minutes **Serving:** 4

Ingredients:

- 4 slices smoked salmon

- 1/2 cup cream cheese

Instructions:

1. Spread a thin layer of cream cheese on each slice of smoked salmon.

2. Roll them up and secure with toothpicks if needed.

3. Serve chilled.

Nutritional Information: Approximately 250 calories, 15g protein, 20g fat, 2g carbs, 0g fiber.

Tips: Add a touch of fresh dill or lemon zest for extra flavor.

8. Prosciutto-Wrapped Melon Bites

Preparation Time: 15 minutes **Serving:** 4

Ingredients:

- 8 slices prosciutto

- 1/2 small cantaloupe or honeydew, cut into bite-sized pieces

Instructions:

1. Wrap each melon bite with a slice of prosciutto.

2. Secure with toothpicks if desired.

3. Serve chilled.

Nutritional Information: Approximately 180 calories, 12g protein, 10g fat, 8g carbs, 1g fiber.

Tips: Choose ripe and sweet melon for a delightful contrast with the salty prosciutto.

9. Egg Yolk Fudge

Cooking Time: 15 minutes (plus chilling time) **Serving:** 6

Ingredients:

- 6 egg yolks

- 1/2 cup unsalted butter

- 1/4 cup powdered erythritol

- 1 teaspoon vanilla extract

Instructions:

1. In a saucepan, melt butter over low heat.

2. Whisk in egg yolks, erythritol, and vanilla extract until well combined.

3. Pour the mixture into a mold and refrigerate until set.

Nutritional Information: Approximately 300 calories, 6g protein, 30g fat, 2g carbs, 0g fiber.

Tips: Use silicone molds for easy removal and different shapes.

10. Chicken Liver Mousse with Bacon "Crackers"

Cooking Time: 30 minutes (plus chilling time) **Serving:** 4

Ingredients:

- 1 cup chicken liver mousse

- 8 slices cooked bacon

Instructions:

1. Spread chicken liver mousse on cooked bacon slices.

2. Roll them up and chill in the refrigerator before slicing.

3. Serve cold.

Nutritional Information: Approximately 350 calories, 18g protein, 30g fat, 2g carbs, 0g fiber.

Tips: Choose a smooth and flavorful chicken liver mousse for the best taste.

MEAL PLANNER JOURNAL

WEEKLY PLANNER WEEK ______________

Monday

Tuesday

Wednesday

Thursday

Friday

Saturday

Sunday

To Do List

- [ ] _______________
- [ ] _______________
- [ ] _______________
- [ ] _______________
- [ ] _______________
- [ ] _______________
- [ ] _______________
- [ ] _______________
- [ ] _______________
- [ ] _______________
- [ ] _______________
- [ ] _______________

Notes

WEEKLY PLANNER

WEEK ______________

Monday

Tuesday

Wednesday

Thursday

Friday

Saturday

Sunday

To Do List

☐ ________________
☐ ________________
☐ ________________
☐ ________________
☐ ________________
☐ ________________
☐ ________________
☐ ________________
☐ ________________
☐ ________________
☐ ________________
☐ ________________

Notes

WEEKLY PLANNER

WEEK _______________

Monday

Tuesday

Wednesday

Thursday

Friday

Saturday

Sunday

To Do List

- [ ]
- [ ]
- [ ]
- [ ]
- [ ]
- [ ]
- [ ]
- [ ]
- [ ]
- [ ]
- [ ]
- [ ]

Notes

WEEKLY PLANNER WEEK ____________

Monday

Tuesday

Wednesday

Thursday

Friday

Saturday

Sunday

To Do List

- [ ]
- [ ]
- [ ]
- [ ]
- [ ]
- [ ]
- [ ]
- [ ]
- [ ]
- [ ]
- [ ]
- [ ]

Notes

WEEKLY PLANNER WEEK _______________

Monday	To Do List

Monday

Tuesday

Wednesday

Thursday

Friday

Saturday

Sunday

To Do List

- [ ] _______________
- [ ] _______________
- [ ] _______________
- [ ] _______________
- [ ] _______________
- [ ] _______________
- [ ] _______________
- [ ] _______________
- [ ] _______________
- [ ] _______________
- [ ] _______________
- [ ] _______________

Notes

____

____

____

____

____

____

WEEKLY PLANNER WEEK _____________

Monday

Tuesday

Wednesday

Thursday

Friday

Saturday

Sunday

To Do List

- ☐ ________________
- ☐ ________________
- ☐ ________________
- ☐ ________________
- ☐ ________________
- ☐ ________________
- ☐ ________________
- ☐ ________________
- ☐ ________________
- ☐ ________________
- ☐ ________________

Notes

WEEKLY PLANNER WEEK _____________

Monday	**To Do List**
	☐ ________________
	☐ ________________
Tuesday	☐ ________________
	☐ ________________
	☐ ________________
Wednesday	☐ ________________
	☐ ________________
	☐ ________________
Thursday	☐ ________________
	☐ ________________
	☐ ________________
Friday	☐ ________________
Saturday	**Notes**
Sunday	

WEEKLY PLANNER WEEK ___________

Monday

Tuesday

Wednesday

Thursday

Friday

Saturday

Sunday

To Do List

☐ ____________________
☐ ____________________
☐ ____________________
☐ ____________________
☐ ____________________
☐ ____________________
☐ ____________________
☐ ____________________
☐ ____________________
☐ ____________________
☐ ____________________
☐ ____________________

Notes

WEEKLY PLANNER

WEEK ________________

Monday	To Do List
Tuesday	☐ ____________
Wednesday	☐ ____________
Thursday	☐ ____________
Friday	☐ ____________
Saturday	Notes
Sunday	

WEEKLY PLANNER WEEK ______________

Monday	To Do List
Tuesday	☐ _______________
Wednesday	☐ _______________
Thursday	☐ _______________
Friday	Notes
Saturday	
Sunday